Blood Sugar Solution Kit Book

The Complete Guide to Managing Your Blood Sugar - Essential Strategies, Recipes, and Tips for Optimal Health

Hephzibah Precious

Copyright Page

Table of Contents

Introduction

I am delighted the Blood Sugar Solution Kit Book found its way into your hands. Whether you are here to take control of your health or seeking answers to some burning questions about blood sugar management, you have come to the right place.

Let's start by understanding why blood sugar regulation is crucial for your overall well-being. Just like a car needs the right type and amount of fuel to run smoothly, the human body requires balanced blood sugar levels to function optimally. From providing energy for daily activities to supporting vital organs like the brain and heart, maintaining stable blood sugar is key to feeling our best every day.

Now, let me address some common misconceptions and myths surrounding blood sugar. You may have heard that all carbohydrates are bad or that sugar is the main culprit behind blood sugar spikes. However, the truth is more nuanced. While it is important to be mindful of your sugar intake, not all carbs are created equal. In fact, whole grains, fruits, and vegetables are part of a healthy diet that supports stable blood sugar levels.

Another myth is that only people with diabetes need to worry about blood sugar. In reality, blood sugar imbalances can affect anyone, regardless of their age or health status. You can take proactive steps to prevent future health issues and maintain vitality throughout your life by understanding how to regulate your blood sugar. So, whether you are looking to optimize your health or simply curious about the science behind blood sugar, this book is your comprehensive guide to managing your blood sugar and achieving optimal wellness. Get ready to empower yourself with essential strategies, delicious recipes, and practical tips for lifelong health.

Chapter 1

The Science Behind Blood Sugar

Understanding the science behind blood sugar is crucial for effectively managing your blood sugar levels and achieving optimal health. In this chapter, we will explore the complex mechanisms that govern blood sugar regulation in the body. You will be better equipped to make informed decisions about your diet, lifestyle, and health if you understand how blood sugar works and the factors that influence its levels.

First in this chapter, I will walk you through the importance of insulin and glucose in maintaining healthy blood sugar levels. Insulin is a hormone produced by the pancreas that helps regulate blood sugar by allowing cells to absorb glucose from the bloodstream.

Glucose, on the other hand, is the primary source of energy for the body and plays a vital role in fueling cellular functions.

We will also explore the impact of imbalanced blood sugar levels on your health. Chronic high blood sugar levels can lead to serious health complications, including type 2 diabetes, cardiovascular disease, and obesity. Conversely, low blood sugar levels can cause symptoms such as fatigue, dizziness, and confusion.

In addition, we will examine the different factors that can influence blood sugar levels, including diet, exercise, stress, and medication. Understanding how these factors affect blood sugar regulation will make you better equipped to make lifestyle choices that promote optimal blood sugar health. Furthermore, I will provide you with practical tips and strategies for managing your blood sugar levels effectively. Whether you are looking to prevent or manage diabetes, lose weight, or simply improve your overall health, the information I will provide you with in this chapter will empower you to take control of your blood sugar and live your best life.

How Blood Sugar Works in the Body

In understanding how blood sugar operates within the body, it is crucial to grasp the complex processes that occur to maintain optimal health. Blood sugar, also known as glucose, serves as the primary source of energy for cells throughout the body. When we consume carbohydrates, they are broken down into glucose during digestion, which then enters the bloodstream. This influx of glucose triggers the release of insulin from the pancreas, a hormone responsible for facilitating the uptake of glucose into cells for energy production.

As glucose enters the cells, it provides the
necessary fuel for different bodily functions,
including muscle contraction, brain activity, and
cellular metabolism. However, it is essential to
maintain a delicate balance of blood sugar
levels to prevent fluctuations that can lead to
health complications. The body can be likened
to a well-coordinated team, with each cell
playing a crucial role in maintaining harmony.
When glucose levels are too high, as seen in
conditions like diabetes, it is similar to an
overabundance of players on the field,
overwhelming the system and disrupting
normal function. On the other hand, low blood
sugar levels can leave cells deprived of energy,
much like a team running out of steam during a
game. To ensure proper regulation of blood
sugar, the body employs a sophisticated
feedback mechanism involving hormones such
as insulin and glucagon. Insulin acts as the key
that unlocks the cells and allows glucose to
enter and be utilized for energy. On the

contrary, glucagon serves as a counter-regulatory hormone that signals the liver to release stored glucose into the bloodstream when levels drop too low.

This delicate balance between insulin and glucagon ensures that blood sugar levels remain within a narrow range, typically between 70 and 120 milligrams per deciliter (mg/dL) in a fasting state. However, several factors can influence these levels, including dietary choices, physical activity, stress, and underlying health conditions. For example, consuming a meal high in refined carbohydrates, such as sugary snacks or processed foods, can cause a rapid spike in blood sugar levels. In response, the pancreas secretes more insulin to help cells absorb the excess glucose, but over time, this can lead to insulin resistance and eventual dysfunction of the insulin-producing cells.

Similarly, engaging in regular physical activity helps to regulate blood sugar levels by increasing insulin sensitivity and promoting the uptake of glucose into muscles for energy. On the other hand, prolonged periods of inactivity can impair insulin function and contribute to insulin resistance.

Stress also plays a significant role in blood sugar regulation, as the body's natural response to stress involves releasing hormones like cortisol, which elevates blood sugar levels. Chronic stress can disrupt this delicate balance and increase the risk of developing insulin resistance and type 2 diabetes.

Impact of insulin and Glucose on Health

Insulin and glucose play vital roles in maintaining our overall health and well-being. Understanding how these two elements interact in our bodies is essential for managing blood sugar levels effectively and preventing complications associated with conditions like diabetes. Insulin, produced by the pancreas, acts as a key that unlocks the cells. This allows glucose to enter and be utilized for energy. When we consume carbohydrates, they are broken down into glucose during digestion and absorbed into the bloodstream. In response, the pancreas releases insulin to regulate the amount of glucose in the blood and facilitate its transport into cells.

One of the key functions of insulin is to help cells absorb glucose from the bloodstream, where it will be used as a source of energy. Without adequate insulin or proper insulin function, glucose cannot enter cells effectively. This will lead to elevated blood sugar levels—a hallmark of diabetes. However, insulin does much more than just regulate blood sugar. It also plays a crucial role in lipid metabolism, protein synthesis, and the storage of excess nutrients. For example, insulin helps convert excess glucose into glycogen—a storage form of glucose found in the liver and muscles. This stored glycogen can be tapped into when energy demands are high, such as during physical activity or periods of fasting.

In addition to its metabolic functions, insulin also has profound effects on other bodily systems. For instance, it promotes the growth and development of tissues, including muscle and fat cells. It also influences the balance of electrolytes in the body and regulates blood pressure by promoting the retention of sodium and water by the kidneys.

Conversely, imbalances in insulin production or function can have serious consequences for health. In individuals with type 1 diabetes, the pancreas produces little to no insulin, resulting in uncontrolled blood sugar levels. On the other hand, type 2 diabetes is characterized by insulin resistance, where cells become less responsive to the effects of insulin, leading to elevated blood sugar levels.

High blood sugar levels, if left unchecked, may lead to a host of complications, including cardiovascular disease, nerve damage, kidney dysfunction, and vision problems. Additionally, persistently elevated insulin levels can contribute to obesity, insulin resistance, and metabolic syndrome—a cluster of conditions that increase the risk of heart disease, stroke, and type 2 diabetes. Therefore, maintaining a delicate balance between insulin and glucose is crucial for optimal health. By adopting a healthy lifestyle that includes regular exercise, a balanced diet, stress management, and adequate sleep, you can support proper insulin function and keep blood sugar levels within a healthy range.

Factors Influencing Blood Sugar Levels

In understanding blood sugar levels, various factors play significant roles. These factors influence how our bodies manage glucose and impact our overall health and well-being. Let's consider some of these crucial factors and how they affect blood sugar regulation:

1. **Dietary Choices**: What you eat directly affects your blood sugar levels. Carbohydrates, especially refined ones like white bread and sugary snacks, often cause a rapid spike in blood sugar levels. On the other hand, fiber-rich foods like fruits, vegetables, and whole grains help stabilize blood sugar by slowing down the absorption of glucose into the bloodstream.

2. **Meal Timing and Frequency**: The timing and frequency of your meals also influence blood sugar levels. Skipping meals or going too long without eating can lead to drops in blood sugar, while consistent meal timing helps maintain stable levels throughout the day. It is essential to eat balanced meals and snacks regularly to keep blood sugar levels steady.

3. **Physical Activity**: Regular exercise is a powerful tool for managing blood sugar levels. Physical activity helps cells absorb glucose from the bloodstream and reduces blood sugar levels. Both aerobic exercise, like walking or cycling, and strength training can improve insulin sensitivity and contribute to better blood sugar control.

4. **Stress Levels**: Stress triggers the release of hormones like cortisol and adrenaline, which can raise blood sugar levels. Chronic stress may lead to persistent elevation of blood sugar, increasing the risk of

developing insulin resistance and type 2 diabetes. Finding ways to manage stress, such as meditation, deep breathing exercises, or engaging in hobbies, is essential for maintaining healthy blood sugar levels.

5. **The Quality of Sleep**: Poor sleep habits disrupt hormone levels and negatively impact blood sugar regulation. Sleep deprivation can lead to insulin resistance and increased appetite, making it harder to control blood sugar levels. Prioritizing good sleep hygiene, such as maintaining a consistent sleep schedule and creating a relaxing bedtime routine, is crucial for overall health and blood sugar management.

6. **Medication and Supplements**: Certain medications and supplements affect blood sugar levels. For example, some medications used to treat high blood pressure or cholesterol may cause blood

sugar fluctuations as a side effect. That is
why it is important to discuss any
medications or supplements with your
healthcare provider to understand their
potential impact on blood sugar and adjust
your treatment plan accordingly.

7. **Underlying Health Conditions**: Certain
   medical conditions, such as thyroid
   disorders and hormonal imbalances
   influence blood sugar levels. Additionally,
   conditions like polycystic ovary syndrome
   (PCOS) and pre-diabetes may affect insulin
   sensitivity and glucose metabolism.
   Managing these underlying health issues is
   crucial for maintaining optimal blood sugar
   control.

By paying attention to these factors and
making proactive lifestyle choices, you can
effectively manage your blood sugar levels and
promote your overall health and well-being. But
let me add this: It is essential to work closely
with your healthcare provider to develop a

personalized plan that addresses your specific needs and goals.

Chapter 2

Assessing Your Blood Sugar Levels

Assessing your blood sugar levels involves more than just checking numbers; it requires a comprehensive understanding of how your body responds to different factors such as food, exercise, and stress. You can make informed decisions to better manage your health and prevent complications associated with imbalanced blood sugar if you have insight about your blood sugar levels. By the end of this chapter, you will have a clearer understanding of how to assess your blood sugar levels effectively and take proactive steps towards achieving optimal health.

I want to emphasize that assessing your blood sugar levels is not about judgment or criticism. It is about empowerment and taking control of your health. No matter where your current blood sugar levels stand, there are always steps you can take to improve and optimize your health outcomes. Whether you are just starting or have been managing your blood sugar for years, there is always room for improvement and growth.

In the next sections of this chapter, you will learn techniques for monitoring blood sugar, interpreting glucose readings, and identifying patterns and trends. By mastering these skills, you will gain valuable insights into your body's response to various factors and empower yourself to make positive changes for better health.

Techniques for Monitoring Blood Sugar

Monitoring your blood sugar levels is essential for managing your health effectively. You will gain valuable insights into how your body responds to food, exercise, and other factors by regularly tracking your glucose levels. Here, I will share different techniques to help you monitor your blood sugar with ease.

1. **Blood Glucose Meters**: These devices are widely used for at-home monitoring of blood sugar levels. To use a glucose meter, you will need a small blood sample obtained by pricking your finger with a lancet. Once you apply the blood to a test strip, insert it into the meter, and in seconds, you will receive a reading of your current glucose level.

2. **Continuous Glucose Monitoring (CGM) Systems**: CGM systems offer real-time monitoring of blood sugar levels throughout

the day. A tiny sensor inserted under the skin measures glucose levels in the interstitial fluid, providing continuous data to a monitor or smartphone app. This technology offers a comprehensive view of blood sugar trends and fluctuations, and allows for more precise management.

3. **Flash Glucose Monitoring**: Similar to CGM systems, flash glucose monitoring involves wearing a sensor on the skin. However, instead of providing continuous readings, users must scan the sensor with a reader device to obtain glucose data. While not as real-time as CGM, flash glucose monitoring still offers valuable insights into blood sugar patterns.

4. **Urine Testing**: Although less common than other methods, urine testing can provide an indication of blood sugar levels. However, it is important to note that urine testing reflects past blood sugar levels rather than current readings. This method is often used

as a supplement to blood glucose monitoring rather than a primary tool.

5. **Smartphone Apps**: With the rise of digital health technologies, many smartphone apps now offer blood sugar tracking capabilities. These apps allow users to input glucose readings manually or sync data from connected devices like glucose meters or CGM systems. Some apps also provide additional features such as meal logging, medication reminders, and data analysis.

6. **Lab Tests**: In addition to at-home monitoring, healthcare providers may recommend periodic lab tests to assess overall blood sugar control. These tests, such as the A1C test, measure average blood glucose levels over a few months, and provides a more comprehensive view of long-term management.

You can stay proactive in managing your blood sugar levels by integrating these monitoring techniques into your routine. Also, consult with your healthcare provider to determine the most appropriate monitoring method for your individual needs. Together, you can develop a personalized monitoring plan to optimize your health and well-being.

Interpreting Glucose Readings

Interpreting glucose readings is crucial for understanding your blood sugar levels and making informed decisions about your health. When you receive your glucose readings, whether from a blood glucose meter or continuous glucose monitor (CGM), it is important to know what these numbers mean and how they relate to your overall well-being.

Glucose readings indicate the concentration of glucose, or sugar, in your bloodstream at a specific time. For those with diabetes or those monitoring their blood sugar for other health reasons, these readings provide valuable insights into how their bodies are processing glucose. The readings are typically expressed in milligrams per deciliter (mg/dL) or millimoles per liter (mmol/L), depending on the measurement system used in your country. In the United States, mg/dL is the standard unit of measurement, while mmol/L is commonly used in other parts of the world.

When interpreting your glucose readings, there are a few key points to consider:

1. **Target Range**: Your healthcare provider will establish a target range for your blood sugar levels based on factors such as your age, overall health, and whether you have diabetes. This range reflects the optimal balance of glucose in your bloodstream for maintaining energy levels and preventing complications.

2. **Normal Levels**: For people without diabetes, normal fasting blood sugar levels

typically range from 70 to 100 mg/dL (3.9 to 5.6 mmol/L). After meals, blood sugar levels may rise temporarily but should return to the normal range within a few hours.

3. **High Blood Sugar (Hyperglycemia)**: Elevated blood sugar levels, known as hyperglycemia, may indicate insulin resistance or insufficient insulin production in individuals with diabetes. Symptoms of hyperglycemia may include increased thirst, frequent urination, fatigue, and blurred vision. If your glucose readings consistently exceed your target range, it is important to consult your healthcare provider to adjust your treatment plan accordingly.

4. **Low Blood Sugar (Hypoglycemia)**: Low blood sugar levels, or hypoglycemia, may occur when there is too much insulin in your bloodstream and cause glucose levels to drop below normal. Symptoms of hypoglycemia may include sweating,

trembling, confusion, and irritability. If your
glucose readings fall below your target
range, it is crucial to consume fast-acting
carbohydrates, such as fruit juice or
glucose tablets, to raise your blood sugar
levels quickly.

5. **Variability**: In addition to individual glucose
    readings, it is essential to consider the
    variability of your blood sugar levels
    throughout the day. Fluctuations in blood
    sugar can be influenced by factors such as
    meals, physical activity, stress, medication,
    and hormonal changes. Keeping a log of
    your glucose readings and noting any
    associated factors will help you identify
    patterns and make adjustments to your
    lifestyle or treatment plan as needed.

Lastly, note that interpreting glucose readings
requires attention to detail and an
understanding of how several factors can
impact blood sugar levels.

Identifying Patterns and Trends

In this section, we delve into the crucial task of identifying patterns and trends in your blood sugar levels. Understanding these patterns will provide you with invaluable insights into your overall health and help you make informed decisions about managing your blood sugar effectively.

One of the key aspects of managing blood sugar is recognizing trends over time. You can identify patterns that may indicate areas of concern or success in your management efforts by tracking your blood sugar levels consistently. These trends can vary from person to person, but common patterns include:

1. **Time of Day**: Pay attention to how your blood sugar levels fluctuate throughout the day. You may notice patterns such

as higher readings after meals or dips during periods of physical activity.

2. **Meal Impact**: Assess how different foods affect your blood sugar levels. Certain foods, especially those high in carbohydrates, may cause spikes in blood sugar, while others may have a more gradual impact.

3. **Physical Activity**: Monitor how exercise influences your blood sugar levels. Regular physical activity can help stabilize blood sugar levels over time, but intense or prolonged exercise may cause fluctuations.

4. **Stress and Emotions**: Recognize the impact of stress, emotions, and other external factors on your blood sugar levels. Stress hormones may raise blood sugar levels, so managing stress is essential for maintaining stability.

Blood sugar levels can vary from day to day, but excessive variability may indicate underlying issues or challenges in management. Analyzing variability involves examining fluctuations in blood sugar levels and identifying potential triggers or contributing factors.

1. **Consistency**: Aim for consistency in your blood sugar readings by following a consistent meal schedule, incorporating regular physical activity, and managing stress effectively.

2. **Identifying Triggers**: Pay attention to factors that may trigger fluctuations in your blood sugar levels, such as certain foods, stressors, medication changes, or illness. Keeping a detailed journal will help you identify patterns and make necessary adjustments.

3. **Consulting Healthcare Professionals:** If you notice significant variability or patterns that concern you, consult with your healthcare provider. They will help you identify underlying issues and

develop a personalized plan for managing your blood sugar effectively.

Tracking your blood sugar levels over time allows you to monitor your progress and evaluate the effectiveness of your management strategies. Regular monitoring and analysis will help you make informed decisions about adjustments to your diet, medication, exercise routine, and lifestyle habits.

I. **Setting Goals**: Establish realistic goals for managing your blood sugar levels based on your individual health needs and preferences. Monitor your progress toward these goals regularly and adjust your approach as needed.

II. **Celebrate Successes**: Celebrate milestones and successes along your journey to better blood sugar management. Recognize the efforts you have made and the progress you have achieved, no matter how small.

III. **Staying Committed**: Stay committed to your blood sugar management plan, even when faced with challenges or setbacks. And don't forget that managing blood sugar is a lifelong journey, and consistency is key to long-term success.

Consistent monitoring, analysis, and adjustment are essential components of successful blood sugar management.

Chapter 3

Lifestyle Strategies for Blood Sugar Control

Lifestyle factors encompass a wide range of habits and behaviors that can significantly impact blood sugar regulation. In this chapter, I will take you through the practical approaches to controlling blood sugar beyond just diet and exercise. While nutrition and physical activity are crucial components of blood sugar management, other lifestyle factors also deserve attention. We'll discuss strategies for optimizing sleep, managing daily routines, and creating a supportive environment for healthy living.

Let's start by discussing the importance of sleep in blood sugar control. Quality sleep is essential for overall health, including metabolic function and blood sugar regulation. Research has shown that inadequate sleep can disrupt hormone levels and lead to insulin resistance and higher blood sugar levels. By prioritizing sleep and establishing healthy sleep habits, you can support your body's natural processes for maintaining optimal blood sugar levels.

Next, we will explore the significance of daily routines in blood sugar management. Consistency is key when it comes to regulating blood sugar levels. By establishing regular meal times, incorporating physical activity into your daily schedule, and managing stress effectively, you can help stabilize your blood sugar throughout the day. We'll discuss practical tips for structuring your day to promote stable blood sugar levels and enhance overall health. With the right knowledge and tools at your disposal, you can take control of your blood sugar and live your best life.

Importance of Diet and Nutrition

Diet and nutrition play a vital role in managing your blood sugar levels and overall health. What you eat directly impacts your body's ability to regulate glucose, insulin, and other essential hormones. By making informed dietary choices, you can effectively manage your blood sugar and reduce the risk of complications associated with diabetes and other metabolic disorders.

One of the key components of a blood sugar-friendly diet is carbohydrate management. Carbohydrates are the primary source of glucose in the body, and they have a direct impact on blood sugar levels. It is important to focus on consuming complex carbohydrates such as whole grains, fruits, vegetables, and legumes, as these foods are rich in fiber, vitamins, and minerals. Fiber slows down the absorption of glucose, preventing rapid spikes in blood sugar levels. In contrast, simple carbohydrates like refined sugars and processed foods may cause sharp increases in blood sugar, leading to energy crashes and cravings. Minimizing the intake of sugary beverages, candies, pastries, and white bread will help stabilize blood sugar levels and promote better overall health.

Another essential aspect of blood sugar control is portion control. Even healthy foods can impact blood sugar if consumed in excessive amounts. You will prevent overeating and keep your blood sugar levels stable throughout the day by paying attention to portion sizes and practicing mindful eating.

More so, meal timing plays a crucial role in blood sugar management. Eating regular, balanced meals and snacks at consistent intervals helps regulate insulin secretion and prevents drastic fluctuations in blood sugar levels. Aim to space your meals evenly throughout the day, with no more than 4-5 hours between each eating occasion.

Furthermore, incorporating healthy fats into your diet will improve blood sugar control and promote satiety. Sources of healthy fats include avocados, nuts, seeds, olive oil, and fatty fish like salmon and mackerel. These fats help slow down the absorption of carbohydrates, preventing rapid spikes in blood sugar and keeping you feeling full and satisfied. Additionally, protein is an essential nutrient for blood sugar management. Including lean protein sources such as chicken, turkey, tofu, eggs, and legumes in your meals can help stabilize blood sugar levels and support muscle growth and repair. Aim to include protein-rich foods in each meal and snack to maintain balanced nutrition throughout the day.

Kindly note that making informed dietary choices is the first step towards achieving

optimal blood sugar control and living a
healthier, happier life.

Effective Exercise Routines

Exercise plays a crucial role in maintaining
optimal health and can significantly impact your
body's ability to regulate blood sugar. You can
improve your insulin sensitivity, reduce blood
sugar spikes, and enhance your overall
well-being by engaging in physical activity.

Regular exercise offers a multitude of benefits
for individuals seeking to control their blood
sugar levels. Firstly, physical activity helps to
improve insulin sensitivity and allows your cells
to more effectively utilize glucose from the
bloodstream. This means that with regular
exercise, your body becomes more efficient at
using insulin to transport glucose into cells,
thereby lowering blood sugar levels.

Furthermore, engaging in exercise promotes
weight management, which is essential for

blood sugar control. Maintaining a healthy weight will reduce insulin resistance and decrease the risk of developing type 2 diabetes. Additionally, exercise has been shown to lower blood pressure, improve cardiovascular health, and enhance mood and mental well-being.

Types of Exercise for Blood Sugar Control

When it comes to choosing the right exercise routine, it is important to find activities that you enjoy and that fit into your lifestyle. So, aim for a combination of aerobic exercise, strength training, and flexibility exercises to reap the maximum benefits for blood sugar control.

- Aerobic exercise, such as walking, jogging, cycling, swimming, or dancing, helps to improve cardiovascular health and burn calories. Aim for at least 150 minutes of moderate-intensity aerobic activity per week, or 75 minutes of vigorous-intensity activity, spread out over several days.

- Strength training exercises, such as lifting weights or using resistance bands, are crucial for building muscle mass and improving overall body composition. Include strength training exercises at least two days a week, targeting major muscle groups like the legs, arms, chest, back, and core.
- Flexibility exercises, such as yoga or stretching, help to improve joint mobility and reduce the risk of injury. Incorporate stretching exercises into your routine on a regular basis to improve flexibility and enhance overall physical performance.

Tips for Incorporating Exercise Into Your Routine

Finding the time and motivation to exercise regularly can be challenging, but with some planning and commitment, it is entirely possible to make physical activity a regular part of your lifestyle.

Here are some tips to help you get started:

1. Schedule exercise sessions into your calendar, just like you would any other appointment. Treat exercise as a non-negotiable part of your day.
2. Find activities that you enjoy and that fit into your schedule. Whether it is going for a walk in the park, taking a dance class, or going for a bike ride, choose activities that you look forward to.
3. Start slowly and gradually increase the intensity and duration of your workouts as your fitness level improves. Remember this:

any amount of physical activity is better than none.

4. Mix it up to prevent boredom and keep your workouts interesting. Try different types of exercise and vary your routine to challenge your body in new ways.

5. Make exercise a social activity by joining a sports team, taking group fitness classes, or exercising with friends or family members. Having a workout buddy will help to keep you accountable and motivated.

As you incorporate exercise into your routine, it is important to monitor your progress and adjust your workouts as needed. Keep track of your activity levels, duration, intensity, and any changes in your blood sugar levels to gauge the effectiveness of your exercise regimen. Consider using a fitness tracker or smartphone app to monitor your daily steps, distance, and calories burned. Keep a journal to record your workouts, including the type of exercise, duration, and any observations or changes in how you feel.

Additionally, be mindful of how exercise affects your blood sugar levels. Monitor your blood sugar before and after exercise, and adjust your carbohydrate intake and insulin dosage as needed to prevent hypoglycemia or hyperglycemia.

Don't forget to consult with your healthcare provider before starting any new exercise program, especially if you have any underlying health conditions or concerns.

Stress Management Techniques

Stress can significantly impact your blood sugar levels, making it crucial to incorporate effective stress management techniques into your daily routine. Chronic stress triggers the release of hormones like cortisol and adrenaline, which may lead to spikes in blood sugar levels over time.

The following are stress management techniques that will help you maintain stable blood sugar levels and improve your overall health.

1. **Deep Breathing Exercises**: Deep breathing exercises are simple but powerful tools for reducing stress and promoting relaxation. Practice deep breathing by inhaling deeply through your nose. This will allow your abdomen to rise as you fill your lungs with air. Hold your breath for a few seconds, then exhale slowly through your mouth, allowing your abdomen to fall. Repeat this process several times, focusing on each breath and allowing yourself to let go of tension with each exhale.

2. **Mindfulness Meditation**: Mindfulness meditation involves paying attention to the

present moment without judgment. To do this, find a quiet and comfortable space where you can sit or lie down comfortably. Close your eyes and focus your attention on your breath, noticing the sensation of each inhale and exhale. If your mind wanders, gently bring your focus back to your breath without criticizing yourself. Regular practice of mindfulness meditation will help reduce stress and improve your ability to manage blood sugar levels.

3. **Progressive Muscle Relaxation**: Progressive muscle relaxation is a technique that involves tensing and relaxing different muscle groups in your body to release tension and promote relaxation. Start by tensing the muscles in your feet and toes for a few seconds, then relax them completely. Move slowly up through your body, tensing and relaxing each muscle group, including your legs, abdomen, chest,

arms, and face. While at it, pay attention to the sensations of tension and relaxation in each muscle group, and allow yourself to let go of stress and tension with each relaxation.

4. **Yoga**: Yoga combines physical postures, breathing exercises, and meditation to promote relaxation and reduce stress. Practicing yoga regularly improves flexibility, strength, and balance, while also calming the mind and reducing stress levels. So, choose gentle yoga poses that focus on stretching and relaxation, such as child's pose, forward fold, and corpse pose. Incorporate deep breathing and mindfulness meditation techniques into your yoga practice for maximum stress-relieving benefits.

5. **Spending Time in Nature**: Spending time in nature has been shown to reduce stress

levels and promote feelings of relaxation and well-being. So, take advantage of opportunities to spend time outdoors, whether it is going for a walk in the park, hiking in the mountains, or simply sitting in your backyard or balcony. Connect with the sights, sounds, and sensations of nature, allowing yourself to let go of stress and tension as you immerse yourself in the natural world.

6. **Engaging in Relaxing Activities**: Engaging in activities that you enjoy and find relaxing will help reduce stress and improve your mood. Whether it is reading a book, listening to music, gardening, or spending time with loved ones, make time for activities that bring you joy and help you unwind. Prioritize self-care and emotional well-being by finding healthy ways to relax and recharge.

Experiment with different techniques to find what works best for you, and make stress management a priority in your overall health plan.

Chapter 4

Nutritional Guidelines for Stable Blood Sugar

When it comes to managing your blood sugar levels effectively, nutrition plays a vital role. What you eat can either help stabilize your blood sugar or send it on a rollercoaster ride. Before we delve into the specifics, it is crucial to understand the impact of food on your blood sugar levels. Every bite you take has the potential to either raise or lower your blood sugar, thereby influencing your overall health and well-being.

In this chapter, we will explore different aspects of nutrition that are essential for managing blood sugar levels effectively. From the types of foods to prioritize to the importance of portion control, you will discover everything you need to know to support stable blood sugar levels and promote your overall wellness.

So, if you are ready to take charge of your health and harness the power of nutrition to manage your blood sugar, let's dive in and explore the nutritional guidelines for stable blood sugar.

Choosing the Right Carbohydrates

When it comes to managing your blood sugar levels, selecting the right carbohydrates is crucial. Not all carbs are created equal, and some can have a significant impact on your blood sugar.

Carbohydrates are one of the three macronutrients, alongside protein and fat, that provide energy for the body. They are found in a wide variety of foods, including fruits, vegetables, grains, legumes, and dairy products. Carbohydrates are broken down into glucose, which is the primary source of fuel for the cells. You must note that not all carbohydrates are metabolized at the same rate or have the same effect on blood sugar levels. Highly processed carbohydrates, such as refined grains and sugary snacks, can cause rapid spikes and crashes in blood sugar, leading to feelings of fatigue and hunger.

On the other hand, complex carbohydrates, such as whole grains, fruits, and vegetables, are digested more slowly, resulting in a gradual and steady release of glucose into the bloodstream. This prevents sudden blood sugar spikes and promotes sustained energy levels.

When selecting carbohydrates for optimal blood sugar management, focus on whole, unprocessed foods that are rich in nutrients and fiber.

Here are some examples of healthy carbohydrate sources to include in your diet:

1. **Whole Grains**: Opt for whole grains such as oats, quinoa, brown rice, and barley, which are rich in fiber and essential nutrients. These grains provide sustained energy and help regulate blood sugar levels.

2. **Fruits**: Choose fresh, whole fruits over fruit juices or dried fruits, which often contain added sugars and lack fiber. Berries, apples, oranges, and kiwi are excellent choices that are low on the glycemic index and high in vitamins and antioxidants.

3. **Vegetables**: Incorporate a variety of colorful vegetables into your meals, including leafy greens, broccoli, carrots, and bell peppers. These nutrient-dense foods are low in calories and carbohydrates. This makes them ideal for blood sugar management.

4. **Legumes**: Beans, lentils, and chickpeas are rich in fiber, protein, and complex carbohydrates. They help stabilize blood sugar levels and promote feelings of fullness and satiety.

Practical Tips for Carb Selection

Here are some practical tips to help you make healthier carbohydrate choices:

i. **Read Labels**: When purchasing packaged foods, check the nutrition label for the total carbohydrate content, as well as the fiber and sugar content. Choose products with higher fiber and lower sugar content.

ii. **Limit Added Sugars**: Be mindful of added sugars in processed foods such as sugary drinks, desserts, and snacks. Opt for unsweetened or naturally sweetened alternatives whenever possible.

iii.   **Focus on Whole Foods**: Base your
meals around whole, minimally
processed foods such as fruits,
vegetables, whole grains, and lean
proteins. These foods provide a wealth
of nutrients and are less likely to cause
blood sugar spikes.

iv.   **Watch Portion Sizes**: Pay attention to
portion sizes to avoid consuming
excessive carbohydrates in one sitting.
You can use measuring cups or visual
cues to help you gauge appropriate
serving sizes.

Incorporating Fiber-rich Foods

Incorporating fiber-rich foods into your diet is essential for maintaining stable blood sugar levels and promoting overall health. Fiber is a type of carbohydrate found in plant-based foods that the body cannot digest. Instead, it passes through the digestive system, and aids in digestion and provides many health benefits.

Fiber helps slow down the absorption of sugar into the bloodstream and prevents spikes in blood sugar levels. Additionally, it promotes satiety and can aid in weight management by keeping you feeling full for longer periods. Including a variety of fiber-rich foods in your diet can help you achieve and maintain optimal blood sugar control. Some examples of fiber-rich foods include fruits, vegetables, whole grains, legumes, nuts, and seeds.

Here are some tips for incorporating these foods into your daily meals:

1. **Start your day with a fiber-rich breakfast**: Choose whole grain cereals or oatmeal topped with fresh fruit and nuts for added fiber. Alternatively, try adding vegetables such as spinach, peppers, or mushrooms to your morning omelet or scramble.

2. **Snack on fruits and vegetables**: Keep a variety of fresh fruits and vegetables on hand for convenient snacking. Apples, berries, carrots, and bell peppers are excellent choices that are high in fiber and low in calories.

3. **Include whole grains in your meals**: Opt for whole grain bread, pasta, rice, and quinoa instead of refined grains. These foods are higher in fiber and provide longer-lasting energy. They will help to stabilize your blood sugar levels throughout the day.

4. **Add legumes to soups, salads, and main dishes**: Beans, lentils, and chickpeas are rich in fiber and protein, making them a nutritious addition to any meal. Try incorporating them into soups, salads, stir-fries, or as a meat substitute in tacos or burgers.

5. **Snack on nuts and seeds**: Almonds, walnuts, chia seeds, and flaxseeds are excellent sources of fiber, healthy fats, and protein. Enjoy them as a snack on their own or sprinkle them over yogurt, oatmeal, or salads for added crunch and nutrition.

Don't forget to drink plenty of water throughout the day, as fiber works best when combined with adequate hydration.

Balancing Macronutrients for Optimal Health

Balancing macronutrients is essential for maintaining stable blood sugar levels and promoting optimal health. Macronutrients refer to carbohydrates, proteins, and fats, each playing a crucial role in fueling our bodies and supporting various bodily functions. Achieving the right balance of these macronutrients can help regulate blood sugar, enhance energy levels, and support overall well-being.

1. **Protein**: Incorporating adequate protein into your diet is vital for blood sugar management. Protein helps slow down the digestion process, preventing rapid spikes in blood sugar levels. Additionally, protein aids in muscle repair and growth, supports immune function, and promotes satiety, helping you feel full and satisfied for longer periods. Sources of protein include lean meats like chicken, turkey, and fish, as well

as plant-based options such as tofu, tempeh, legumes, and nuts.

- Example: Enjoy a grilled chicken breast paired with steamed vegetables for a balanced meal that provides protein, vitamins, and minerals without causing significant fluctuations in blood sugar levels.

2. **Fats**: Contrary to popular belief, incorporating healthy fats into your diet can actually support blood sugar control and overall health. Healthy fats, such as those found in avocados, nuts, seeds, and olive oil, help slow down the absorption of carbohydrates, leading to more stable blood sugar levels. Additionally, fats play a crucial role in hormone production, brain function, and the absorption of fat-soluble vitamins like A, D, E, and K.

- Example: Add a handful of walnuts or almonds to your morning oatmeal or yogurt for a dose of healthy fats that will help stabilize blood sugar levels and keep you feeling full until your next meal.

Achieving the right balance of macronutrients can be achieved by following a well-rounded and varied diet that includes a combination of protein, healthy fats, and carbohydrates. Experiment with different food combinations and pay attention to how your body responds to find the optimal balance for your individual needs. Additionally, consider consulting with a registered dietitian or nutritionist for personalized guidance and support in creating a balanced meal plan tailored to your blood sugar goals and overall health objectives.

Chapter 5

Meal Planning and Recipes

Meal planning is not just about what you eat, but also when you eat it. Balancing carbohydrates, proteins, and fats in your meals can help regulate blood sugar levels throughout the day. This chapter provides practical strategies to create balanced meals that support blood sugar stability.

Additionally, we explore recipes tailored to promote blood sugar health. These recipes are designed to be both delicious and nutritious, making it easier for you to stick to your dietary goals. Whether you're cooking for yourself or your family, these recipes offer a variety of options to suit different tastes and preferences.

By incorporating the tips and recipes outlined in this chapter into your daily routine, you can take proactive steps towards managing your blood sugar and achieving optimal health. Let's get started on this journey to better blood sugar control and improved overall wellness.

Sample Meal Plans for Various Dietary Preferences

Meal planning is a crucial aspect of managing blood sugar levels effectively. In this section, I will provide sample meal plans tailored to different dietary preferences.

Low-Carb Meal Plan:

- **Breakfast**: Scrambled eggs with spinach and avocado.
- **Snack**: Mixed nuts or sliced cucumber with hummus.
- **Lunch**: Grilled chicken salad with mixed greens, tomatoes, and olive oil dressing.

- **Snack**: Greek yogurt with berries.
- **Dinner**: Baked salmon with roasted broccoli and quinoa.

Mediterranean Meal Plan:

- **Breakfast**: Greek yogurt with honey and walnuts.
- **Snack**: Whole fruit such as an apple or pear.
- **Lunch**: Mediterranean quinoa salad with feta cheese, olives, and cherry tomatoes.
- **Snack**: Hummus with whole grain crackers.
- **Dinner**: Grilled shrimp with roasted vegetables and whole wheat couscous.

Plant-Based Meal Plan:

- **Breakfast**: Overnight oats made with almond milk, chia seeds, and sliced fruit.
- **Snack**: Carrot sticks with tahini dip.

- **Lunch**: Lentil soup with a side of mixed greens salad.
- **Snack**: Air-popped popcorn seasoned with nutritional yeast.
- **Dinner**: Stir-fried tofu with mixed vegetables and brown rice.

Paleo Meal Plan:

- **Breakfast**: Bacon and vegetable frittata.
- **Snack**: Celery sticks with almond butter.
- **Lunch**: Grilled steak salad with avocado and balsamic vinaigrette.
- **Snack**: Beef jerky or turkey slices.
- **Dinner**: Baked chicken thighs with roasted sweet potatoes and asparagus.

Flexitarian Meal Plan:

- **Breakfast:** Whole grain toast with mashed avocado and a poached egg.
- **Snack**: Cottage cheese with pineapple chunks.

- **Lunch**: Quinoa and black bean bowl with avocado, salsa, and cilantro.
- **Snack**: Edamame or roasted chickpeas.
- **Dinner**: Stir-fried shrimp with mixed vegetables and cauliflower rice.

These sample meal plans are designed to provide balanced nutrition while keeping blood sugar levels stable. Remember to adjust portion sizes and food choices based on your individual preferences and dietary needs. Additionally, consult with a healthcare professional or registered dietitian for personalized guidance and support.

Delicious and Nutritious Recipes for Breakfast, Lunch, Dinner, and Snacks

In this section, I will share a variety of delicious and nutritious recipes for breakfast, lunch, dinner, and snacks. I have carefully put together these recipes to help you manage your blood sugar levels while enjoying flavorful and satisfying meals.

Breakfast Recipes:

1. **Avocado and Egg Breakfast Bowl**: Start your day with a power-packed meal by combining sliced avocado, cooked quinoa, and a poached egg. Sprinkle with a dash of black pepper and a drizzle of olive oil for added flavor.

2. **Greek Yogurt Parfait**: Layer Greek yogurt with fresh berries, chopped nuts, and a

sprinkle of cinnamon for a protein-rich and satisfying breakfast option.

3. **Oatmeal with Berries and Almonds**: Cook rolled oats with almond milk and top with fresh berries and chopped almonds for a hearty and nutritious breakfast that will keep you full until lunchtime.

Lunch Recipes:

1. **Quinoa Salad with Grilled Chicken:** Toss cooked quinoa with mixed greens, cherry tomatoes, cucumber slices, and grilled chicken breast. Drizzle with a balsamic vinaigrette for a light and satisfying lunch option.

2. **Salmon and Avocado Wrap**: Fill a whole-grain wrap with grilled salmon, sliced avocado, shredded lettuce, and diced tomatoes. Roll it up and enjoy a delicious and nutritious lunch on the go.

3. **Vegetable Stir-Fry with Tofu:** Stir-fry a mix of colorful vegetables such as bell peppers,

broccoli, and snap peas with cubed tofu in a light soy sauce. Serve over brown rice for a healthy and flavorful lunch.

Dinner Recipes:

1. **Baked Cod with Roasted Vegetables**: Season cod fillets with lemon juice, garlic, and herbs, then bake until flaky. Serve with a side of roasted vegetables such as carrots, Brussels sprouts, and sweet potatoes for a satisfying and nutritious dinner.

2. **Turkey and Quinoa Stuffed Bell Peppers**: Stuff halved bell peppers with a mix of cooked ground turkey, quinoa, diced tomatoes, and spices. Bake until tender and serve for a flavorful and protein-packed dinner option.

3. **Vegetable and Lentil Curry**: Simmer lentils with a mix of vegetables such as cauliflower, carrots, and spinach in a flavorful curry sauce made with coconut

milk and spices. Serve over brown rice for a comforting and nutritious dinner.

Snack Recipes:

1. **Apple Slices with Peanut Butter**: Slice an apple and serve with a tablespoon of natural peanut butter for a satisfying and protein-rich snack that will keep your blood sugar levels stable between meals.

2. **Greek Yogurt with Almonds and Honey**: Enjoy a serving of Greek yogurt topped with chopped almonds and a drizzle of honey for a delicious and nutritious snack option.

3. **Vegetable Sticks with Hummus**: Cut up raw vegetables such as carrots, celery, and bell peppers and serve with a side of hummus for a crunchy and satisfying snack that's packed with fiber and nutrients.

These recipes are just a starting point for creating delicious and nutritious meals that support healthy blood sugar levels. Feel free to experiment with different ingredients and flavors to find what works best for you. And remember to focus on whole, unprocessed foods and prioritize lean proteins, healthy fats, and fiber-rich carbohydrates for optimal blood sugar control.

Tips for Dining Out While Managing Blood Sugar

When dining out, managing blood sugar levels can be a challenge, but with the right strategies, you can still enjoy meals while keeping your health in check.

Here are some tips to help you navigate restaurant menus and make smart choices:

1. **Plan Ahead**: Before heading to a restaurant, take a look at the menu online if possible. This way, you can identify healthier options and plan your meal accordingly. Look for dishes that are grilled, baked, or steamed rather than fried, and opt for dishes that include lean proteins, vegetables, and whole grains.

2. **Watch Portion Sizes**: Restaurants often serve larger portions than what is recommended for maintaining stable blood sugar levels. Consider sharing a meal with

a friend or family member, or ask for a half portion or a to-go box to save half of your meal for later. This can help prevent overeating and keep your blood sugar in check.

3. **Choose Wisely**: When ordering, focus on filling your plate with nutrient-dense foods. Start with a salad or broth-based soup to help fill you up without adding too many calories or carbohydrates. For your main dish, opt for lean proteins such as grilled chicken or fish, and ask for steamed or roasted vegetables as a side.

4. **Be Mindful of Hidden Sugars**: Keep an eye out for hidden sugars in sauces, dressings, and marinades. These can quickly add up and spike your blood sugar levels. Ask for sauces and dressings on the side so you can control how much you use, or choose dishes that are prepared without added sugars.

5. **Limit Alcohol Intake**: Alcohol affects blood sugar levels and may interfere with your body's ability to regulate glucose. If you choose to drink alcohol while dining out, do so in moderation and opt for lower-sugar options such as dry wines or spirits mixed with soda water.

6. **Stay Hydrated**: Drinking water throughout your meal can help you feel full and prevent overeating. It can also help prevent dehydration, which can contribute to fluctuations in blood sugar levels. Limit sugary beverages such as soda and fruit juice, and opt for water or unsweetened tea instead.

7. **Ask Questions**: Don't be afraid to ask your server about how dishes are prepared or if substitutions can be made to accommodate your dietary needs. Many restaurants are willing to make modifications to dishes to meet your preferences, such as substituting vegetables for rice or potatoes.

8. **Listen to Your Body**: Pay attention to how different foods affect your blood sugar levels and how you feel after eating. If you notice that certain foods cause your blood sugar to spike or leave you feeling sluggish, try to avoid them in the future. Trust your body's signals and make choices that support your health and well-being.

You can enjoy dining out while managing your blood sugar levels effectively by following these tips.

Chapter 6

Supplements and Herbs for Blood Sugar Support

This chapter addresses supplements and herbs that provide valuable support. As you navigate through the options available, it is essential to understand the potential benefits and considerations when incorporating supplements and herbs into your routine. From vitamins and minerals to botanical extracts, these natural remedies offer a complementary approach to traditional methods of blood sugar management.

I will walk you through the role of supplements and herbs in supporting blood sugar health and provide you with valuable insights and practical tips to optimize their effectiveness. Whether you are looking to enhance insulin sensitivity, reduce glucose fluctuations, or improve overall metabolic function, this chapter will equip you with the knowledge and tools necessary to make informed decisions about your health.

Let's uncover the science behind these natural remedies and learn how they play a valuable role in blood sugar management.

Overview of Supplements and Their Role in Blood Sugar Management

Supplements play a crucial role in managing blood sugar levels. In this section, I will provide an overview of different supplements and their significance in blood sugar management.

1. **Vitamin D**: This essential nutrient has been linked to improved insulin sensitivity. This makes it a valuable supplement for those looking to regulate blood sugar levels. Research suggests that maintaining adequate vitamin D levels may reduce the

risk of developing type 2 diabetes. Incorporating a vitamin D supplement into your routine, especially if you have low levels, will be beneficial for overall health and blood sugar control.

2. **Magnesium**: Magnesium is involved in over 300 biochemical reactions in the body, including glucose metabolism. Studies have shown that magnesium deficiency is associated with insulin resistance and impaired glucose tolerance. You can support proper insulin function and enhance blood sugar regulation by supplementing with magnesium. Look for magnesium citrate or glycinate forms for better absorption.

3. **Chromium**: Chromium is a trace mineral that plays a role in insulin action and glucose metabolism. It helps enhance the effectiveness of insulin, allowing for better glucose uptake by cells. Supplementing with chromium has been shown to improve

insulin sensitivity and lower fasting blood sugar levels in persons with diabetes or insulin resistance.

4. **Alpha-Lipoic Acid (ALA)**: ALA is a powerful antioxidant that helps protect cells from damage caused by oxidative stress. It has been studied for its potential benefits in improving insulin sensitivity and reducing insulin resistance. ALA may also help lower blood sugar levels by increasing glucose uptake in cells and improving insulin signaling pathways.

5. **Berberine**: Berberine is a compound extracted from various plants, including goldenseal and barberry. It has been used in traditional medicine for centuries and has shown promising results in improving blood sugar control. Berberine works by activating an enzyme called AMP-activated protein kinase (AMPK), which helps regulate glucose metabolism. Studies have demonstrated that berberine

supplementation significantly reduce blood sugar levels and improve insulin sensitivity.

6. **Fish Oil**: Omega-3 fatty acids found in fish oil have anti-inflammatory properties and may help improve insulin sensitivity. Supplementing with fish oil can also support heart health and reduce the risk of cardiovascular complications associated with diabetes. Look for high-quality fish oil supplements that provide adequate amounts of EPA and DHA.

7. **Probiotics**: Gut health plays a crucial role in overall health, including blood sugar regulation. Probiotics, beneficial bacteria found in fermented foods and supplements, can help maintain a healthy balance of gut flora and improve metabolic health. Research suggests that probiotic supplementation may reduce fasting blood sugar levels and improve insulin sensitivity in individuals with diabetes.

When incorporating supplements into your regimen, it's essential to consult with a healthcare professional to ensure they are safe and appropriate for your individual needs. Additionally, it is important to remember that supplements should complement, not replace, a healthy diet and lifestyle.

Herbal Remedies and Their Potential Benefits

Herbal remedies have long been utilized for their potential benefits in managing blood sugar levels. These natural alternatives offer a variety of compounds that may support glucose regulation and overall health.

The following are some of the most promising herbs for blood sugar support, along with their potential benefits.

1. **Cinnamon**: Cinnamon is a popular spice known for its sweet flavor and aromatic

scent. It contains compounds like cinnamaldehyde and cinnamic acid, which have been studied for their potential to improve insulin sensitivity and lower blood sugar levels. Incorporating cinnamon into your diet may help regulate glucose metabolism and reduce the risk of developing insulin resistance. You can sprinkle cinnamon on oatmeal, yogurt, or add it to smoothies for a flavorful boost.

2. **Fenugreek**: Fenugreek is an herb commonly used in Indian cuisine and traditional medicine. It contains soluble fiber and compounds like trigonelline, which may help improve insulin sensitivity and reduce fasting blood sugar levels. Research suggests that fenugreek supplementation can lead to significant improvements in glycemic control, making it a valuable addition to your blood sugar management routine. You can consume fenugreek seeds

as a spice, brew them into a tea, or take them in supplement form.

3. **Ginseng**: Ginseng is a medicinal herb with a long history of use in traditional Chinese medicine. It contains bioactive compounds called ginsenosides, which have been shown to improve insulin sensitivity and enhance glucose uptake in cells. Studies suggest that ginseng supplementation may help lower fasting blood sugar levels and improve HbA1c levels in individuals with type 2 diabetes. You can enjoy ginseng tea or take it in supplement form to support blood sugar regulation.

4. **Bitter Melon**: Bitter melon, also known as bitter gourd or Momordica charantia, is a tropical fruit that has been used in traditional medicine for its potential health benefits. It contains compounds like charantin, which may help improve insulin secretion and glucose utilization in the body. Research indicates that bitter melon

supplementation can lead to reductions in fasting blood sugar levels and improvements in insulin sensitivity. You can add bitter melon into your diet by cooking it as a vegetable or juicing it for a refreshing beverage.

5. **Berberine**: Berberine is a bioactive compound found in several plants, including goldenseal, Oregon grape, and barberry. It has been studied extensively for its potential to lower blood sugar levels and improve insulin sensitivity. Berberine works by activating AMP-activated protein kinase (AMPK), a key enzyme involved in glucose metabolism. Research suggests that berberine supplementation can lead to significant reductions in fasting blood sugar levels and HbA1c levels in individuals with type 2 diabetes. You can take berberine supplements to support blood sugar control and overall metabolic health.

Incorporating these herbal remedies into your blood sugar solution kit will provide additional support for managing your glucose levels and promoting overall health. However, you should consult with your healthcare provider before starting any new supplement regimen, especially if you are taking medications or have underlying health conditions. By combining these natural alternatives with a healthy diet, regular exercise, and lifestyle modifications, you can take proactive steps towards optimal blood sugar management and long-term wellness.

Precautions and Considerations When Using Supplements

When using supplements to support blood sugar management, it is crucial to be aware of potential precautions and considerations to ensure their safe and effective use.

Below are some important points to keep in mind:

1. **Consult with a Healthcare Professional**: Before starting any new supplement regimen, it is important to consult with a healthcare professional, such as a doctor or registered dietitian. They can provide personalized guidance based on your individual health needs and medication regimen.

2. **Quality and Purity**: When selecting supplements, opt for reputable brands that adhere to strict quality control standards.

Look for products that have been third-party tested for purity and potency to ensure that you are getting a safe and effective product.

3. **Dosage Considerations**: Pay attention to recommended dosage guidelines provided by the manufacturer. Taking more than the recommended dose of certain supplements may lead to adverse effects or interactions with medications. So, start with the lowest effective dose and gradually increase as needed, under the guidance of a healthcare professional.

4. **Potential Interactions**: Be aware of potential interactions between supplements and medications you may be taking. Some supplements may interfere with the absorption or effectiveness of certain medications, so it is important to discuss potential interactions with your healthcare provider.

5. **Monitoring Blood Sugar Levels**: Keep track of your blood sugar levels regularly,

especially when starting a new supplement regimen. This will help you monitor the effects of the supplements on your blood sugar levels and make any necessary adjustments to your treatment plan.

6. **Adverse Effects**: Pay attention to any adverse effects or symptoms that may arise after starting a new supplement. Common side effects of certain supplements include gastrointestinal discomfort, allergic reactions, and changes in blood pressure. If you experience any adverse effects, discontinue use and consult with a healthcare professional.

7. **Safety Precautions**: Store supplements out of reach of children and pets, and follow storage instructions provided by the manufacturer. Additionally, be cautious when purchasing supplements online and ensure that you are buying from reputable sources to avoid counterfeit or adulterated products.

8. **Long-Term Use**: Consider the long-term implications of supplement use and whether it aligns with your overall health goals. While some supplements may provide short-term benefits for blood sugar management, it is important to prioritize sustainable lifestyle changes for long-term health and wellness.

Chapter 7

Blood Sugar Management for Special Populations

There are specialized strategies for managing blood sugar in unique circumstances. So, whether you are navigating dietary restrictions, incorporating exercise into a busy schedule, or dealing with the challenges of everyday life, this section provides targeted guidance to support your blood sugar goals. If you understand the nuances of blood sugar management for special populations, you can empower yourself to make informed choices and prioritize your health. Through practical tips and evidence-based recommendations I will provide you with in this chapter, you will gain valuable insights into optimizing blood sugar levels for enhanced well-being and vitality.

Blood Sugar Considerations During Pregnancy

During pregnancy, managing blood sugar becomes paramount for both the mother's and the baby's health. Fluctuations in blood sugar levels may impact fetal development and increase the risk of complications during pregnancy and delivery. Therefore, it is crucial for expectant mothers to prioritize blood sugar control throughout each trimester.

Maintaining stable blood sugar levels is essential for the overall health and well-being of both the mother and the developing fetus. High blood sugar levels, especially during the early stages of pregnancy, may increase the risk of birth defects and other complications. Conversely, low blood sugar levels can lead to hypoglycemia, which may pose risks to the baby's health.

1. Monitoring Blood Sugar Levels

Regular monitoring of blood sugar levels is vital
for pregnant women with gestational diabetes
or pre-existing diabetes. This can be done
through self-monitoring using a glucometer or
continuous glucose monitoring (CGM) devices.
Expectant mothers can identify patterns and
make necessary adjustments to their diet and
lifestyle by tracking blood sugar levels
throughout the day.

2. Nutritional Guidelines for Blood Sugar Management

Following a balanced diet is key to controlling
blood sugar levels during pregnancy.
Emphasize foods with a low glycemic index,
such as whole grains, fruits, vegetables, lean
proteins, and healthy fats. Avoiding sugary
snacks and beverages is crucial for preventing
spikes in blood sugar levels. Incorporating
fiber-rich foods into meals will help stabilize
blood sugar levels and promote overall
digestive health.

3. **Meal Planning and Snacking**

Planning meals and snacks ahead of time helps pregnant women maintain stable blood sugar levels throughout the day. So, aim for three balanced meals and two to three snacks per day, spaced evenly to prevent large fluctuations in blood sugar. Opt for snacks that combine carbohydrates with protein or healthy fats to provide sustained energy without causing rapid spikes in blood sugar.

4. **Exercise and Physical Activity**

Engaging in regular physical activity is beneficial for both maternal and fetal health during pregnancy. Moderate-intensity exercise, such as walking, swimming, or prenatal yoga, can help improve insulin sensitivity and regulate blood sugar levels. However, it is essential to consult with your doctor before starting any exercise program during pregnancy to ensure safety and appropriateness.

5. **Medication and Insulin Therapy**

Some pregnant women may require medication or insulin therapy to manage their blood sugar levels effectively. Oral medications for diabetes management may need to be adjusted or discontinued during pregnancy, as they can potentially harm the developing fetus. Insulin therapy is often the preferred treatment option for pregnant women with diabetes, as it does not cross the placenta and is considered safe for both mother and baby.

6. **Regular Prenatal Care**

Regular prenatal visits are essential for monitoring blood sugar levels, fetal growth, and overall maternal health throughout pregnancy. Healthcare providers will perform routine blood tests to assess blood sugar control and may recommend additional screenings or interventions as needed. Open communication between the expectant mother and her healthcare team is crucial for optimizing pregnancy outcomes and ensuring the best possible care for both mother and baby.

By following these guidelines and working closely with their doctors, expectant mothers can effectively manage their blood sugar levels during pregnancy and promote the health and well-being of themselves and their babies. Lastly, remember, maintaining stable blood sugar levels is a priority for a healthy pregnancy and delivery.

Managing Blood Sugar in Children and Adolescents

Managing blood sugar in children and adolescents is crucial for their overall health and well-being. As they grow and develop, their bodies undergo many changes that can affect their blood sugar levels.

First and foremost, let me emphasize the importance of a healthy diet for children and adolescents. Encouraging them to consume balanced meals that include plenty of fruits, vegetables, whole grains, and lean proteins will stabilize their blood sugar levels. Avoiding sugary snacks and beverages is also key to maintaining steady glucose levels throughout the day.

Regular physical activity is another crucial component of managing blood sugar in children and adolescents. Encouraging them to engage in at least 60 minutes of moderate to vigorous exercise each day will improve their insulin sensitivity and regulate blood sugar levels. Activities such as biking, swimming, and playing sports are excellent options for keeping kids active and healthy. In addition to diet and exercise, it is important to monitor children's and adolescents' blood sugar levels regularly. This can be done using a blood glucose meter, which allows parents and caregivers to track their child's glucose levels and make any necessary adjustments to their treatment plan. Keeping a log of blood sugar readings can help identify patterns and trends over time.

It is also important to educate children and adolescents about the importance of managing their blood sugar levels and how to do so effectively. Teaching them about the role of insulin in the body and how certain foods and activities can impact their blood sugar levels will empower them to take control of their health from a young age. In some cases, children and adolescents may require medication or insulin therapy to help manage their blood sugar levels. It is important for parents and caregivers to work closely with their child's healthcare team to develop a treatment plan that meets their individual needs and ensures optimal blood sugar control.

Overall, managing blood sugar in children and adolescents requires a comprehensive approach that includes healthy eating, regular physical activity, monitoring blood sugar levels, and education. Are you a parent or caregiver? You can set your children up for a lifetime of good health by taking proactive steps to promote blood sugar health from a young age.

Tips for Seniors and individuals with Specific Health Conditions

As we age or face certain health challenges, managing blood sugar becomes even more crucial for maintaining overall well-being. In this section, I have provided tailored tips for seniors and individuals with specific health conditions to effectively manage their blood sugar levels and promote optimal health.

Seniors:

1. **Prioritize Whole Foods:** As we age, our bodies may become more sensitive to fluctuations in blood sugar. Focus on consuming whole, nutrient-dense foods such as fruits, vegetables, lean proteins, and whole grains. These foods provide essential vitamins, minerals, and fiber while minimizing spikes in blood sugar.

2. **Stay Active**: Regular physical activity is key to managing blood sugar levels, improving insulin sensitivity, and maintaining overall health. Engage in activities that you enjoy and are suitable for your fitness level, such as walking, swimming, or tai chi. Aim for at least 30 minutes of moderate-intensity exercise most days of the week.

3. **Monitor Medications**: Seniors often take multiple medications, some of which may affect blood sugar levels. It's essential to monitor blood sugar closely when starting new medications or making changes to existing ones. Consult with your doctor if you notice any significant changes in your blood sugar readings.

4. **Stay Hydrated**: Dehydration can exacerbate fluctuations in blood sugar levels, especially in older adults. Make sure to drink plenty of water throughout the day

to stay hydrated and support optimal blood
sugar regulation.

5. **Get Adequate Sleep**: Quality sleep is
   crucial for overall health and blood sugar
   management. Aim for 7-9 hours of
   uninterrupted sleep each night to support
   optimal metabolic function and hormone
   regulation.

Individuals with Specific Health Conditions:

1. Diabetes:

i. Follow a personalized meal plan tailored
   to your specific dietary needs and blood
   sugar goals.

ii. Monitor blood sugar levels regularly and
    adjust medication dosages as needed in
    consultation with your healthcare
    provider.

iii. Incorporate stress-reduction techniques
     such as meditation or deep breathing

exercises to help manage blood sugar
levels.

iv. Stay informed about the latest
advancements in diabetes management
and treatment options.

2. Heart Disease:

i. Choose heart-healthy foods that are
also low in added sugars and refined
carbohydrates, such as fruits,
vegetables, whole grains, and lean
proteins.

ii. Aim to achieve and maintain a healthy
weight through a balanced diet and
regular physical activity.

iii. Monitor blood pressure and cholesterol
levels regularly, as these factors can
impact blood sugar control.

iv. Quit smoking and limit alcohol
consumption to reduce the risk of
cardiovascular complications.

3. Kidney Disease:

i.   Limit intake of foods high in potassium, phosphorus, and sodium, as these nutrients can affect kidney function and blood sugar levels.

ii.   Work closely with a registered dietitian to develop a kidney-friendly meal plan that also supports optimal blood sugar control.

iii. Stay hydrated by drinking plenty of water, but consult with your healthcare provider about appropriate fluid intake based on your individual needs.

iv.   Monitor kidney function regularly through blood tests and follow your healthcare provider's recommendations for managing kidney disease and blood sugar levels.

Seniors and individuals with specific health conditions can effectively manage their blood sugar levels and improve their overall health and well-being by implementing these tailored tips and strategies. Meanwhile, remember to consult with your doctor before making any significant changes to your diet, exercise routine, or medication regimen.

Chapter 8

Troubleshooting Common Challenges

This chapter addresses the different challenges that may arise on your journey to managing your blood sugar effectively. As you navigate the complexities of blood sugar control, it is important to be prepared for potential challenges that may arise along the way. It is when you understand how to troubleshoot common issues that you can stay on track towards achieving optimal blood sugar health.

Throughout this chapter, I provide you with practical strategies and solutions to help you overcome hurdles and maintain steady progress towards your goals. From addressing dietary dilemmas to navigating lifestyle adjustments, you will have the tools and insights needed to tackle any roadblocks you may encounter.

Now, let's dive in and explore how to overcome common challenges and continue on your path to optimal blood sugar management.

Dealing with Blood Sugar Fluctuations

Managing blood sugar fluctuations is crucial for maintaining optimal health and preventing complications associated with conditions like diabetes. Fluctuations in blood sugar levels can occur due to various factors, including diet, exercise, stress, medications, and underlying health conditions. In this section, we will explore effective strategies for dealing with blood sugar fluctuations and maintaining stability.

Below are some effective strategies for dealing with blood sugar fluctuations:

1. Monitor Your Blood Sugar Regularly

Regular monitoring of your blood sugar levels is essential for understanding how your body responds to different foods, activities, and medications. Use a reliable blood glucose meter to check your levels as recommended by your healthcare provider.

2. Follow a Consistent Meal Plan

Consistency in meal timing and composition can help stabilize blood sugar levels throughout the day. Aim to eat balanced meals that include a combination of carbohydrates, protein, and healthy fats. Choose high-fiber foods like fruits, vegetables, whole grains, and legumes, which can slow the absorption of glucose into the bloodstream. Avoid skipping meals or consuming large amounts of refined carbohydrates, as these may lead to rapid spikes and crashes in blood sugar.

3. Incorporate Physical Activity into Your Routine

Regular exercise is an effective way to improve insulin sensitivity and regulate blood sugar levels. Engage in moderate-intensity activities such as brisk walking, cycling, swimming, or dancing for at least 30 minutes most days of the week. Find activities that you enjoy and can easily incorporate into your daily routine. Remember to check your blood sugar before and after exercise, as physical activity can affect your levels.

4. Manage Stress Effectively

Chronic stress have a significant impact on blood sugar levels by triggering the release of stress hormones like cortisol and adrenaline. Practice stress-reducing techniques such as deep breathing, meditation, yoga, or tai chi to promote relaxation and mental well-being. Prioritize self-care activities and seek support from friends, family, or a counselor if you're feeling overwhelmed.

5. Stay Hydrated

Drinking an adequate amount of water is important for maintaining hydration and supporting overall health, including blood sugar regulation. Aim to drink at least 8-10 glasses of water per day, or more if you're physically active or live in a hot climate. Limit your intake of sugary beverages and alcohol, as these can contribute to fluctuations in blood sugar and dehydration.

6. Adjust Your Medications as Needed

If you are taking medications to manage your blood sugar, work closely with your healthcare provider to adjust your dosage as needed based on your blood glucose readings and lifestyle changes. Never make changes to your medication regimen without consulting a healthcare professional, as this can lead to dangerous fluctuations in blood sugar levels.

7. Seek Immediate Medical Attention for Severe Fluctuations

If you experience severe fluctuations in blood sugar levels accompanied by symptoms such as dizziness, confusion, weakness, or loss of consciousness, seek medical attention immediately. These could be signs of a serious medical emergency requiring prompt treatment.

By implementing these strategies and staying proactive in managing your blood sugar levels, you will minimize fluctuations and maintain better overall health.

Overcoming Plateaus in Progress

Overcoming plateaus in progress can be a frustrating challenge when managing your blood sugar levels. Despite your best efforts, you may find yourself stuck at a certain point without seeing further improvement. However, it is important to remember that plateaus are a normal part of any health journey and can be overcome with the right strategies and mindset.

One effective approach to overcoming plateaus is to reassess your current routine and make necessary adjustments. This may involve revisiting your dietary habits, exercise regimen, or stress management techniques. By identifying areas where you may have become complacent or where improvements can be made, you can jumpstart your progress and break through the plateau.

In terms of diet, it is crucial to evaluate the types and quantities of food you are consuming. Are you still following a balanced diet rich in fiber, lean protein, and healthy fats? Are you monitoring your carbohydrate intake and choosing complex carbohydrates over refined sugars? Sometimes, making small changes such as swapping out processed snacks for whole foods or reducing portion sizes can make a significant difference in blood sugar control.

Additionally, consider incorporating more variety into your meals to prevent boredom and keep your body guessing. Experiment with new recipes and ingredients to keep things fresh and exciting. This not only helps prevent plateaus but also ensures that you are getting a wide range of nutrients to support overall health.

When it comes to exercise, plateau-breaking strategies may involve increasing the intensity or duration of your workouts. If you have been doing the same routine for a while, your body may have adapted to it, resulting in diminished returns. Try incorporating high-intensity interval training (HIIT) or resistance training to challenge your muscles and boost your metabolism.

It is also essential to pay attention to your stress levels and overall lifestyle habits. Chronic stress can negatively impact blood sugar levels and hinder progress towards your goals. Consider incorporating relaxation techniques such as meditation, deep breathing exercises, or yoga into your daily routine to help manage stress effectively. In addition to making adjustments to your diet, exercise, and stress management, seeking support from healthcare professionals or a support group can provide valuable guidance and encouragement. They may offer personalized advice based on your individual needs and help you stay motivated during challenging times.

Emotional and Psychological Aspects of Blood Sugar Management

Managing blood sugar is not just about what you eat or how much you exercise; it also involves addressing the emotional and psychological aspects that can impact your journey to optimal health. Stress, anxiety, and other emotions may have a significant impact on blood sugar levels. This makes it vital to take care of your mental well-being alongside your physical health.

Here are strategies for coping with the emotional and psychological challenges of blood sugar management:

1. **Understanding the Connection Between Emotions and Blood Sugar**: It is essential

to recognize that emotions such as stress, anxiety, and depression can affect blood sugar levels. When you're stressed or anxious, your body releases hormones like cortisol and adrenaline, which can cause blood sugar to rise. Additionally, emotional eating, where you turn to food for comfort or distraction, leads to unhealthy eating habits and blood sugar imbalances.

2. **Practicing Stress Management Techniques:** One of the most effective ways to address the emotional aspects of blood sugar management is by incorporating stress management techniques into your daily routine. This may include activities such as meditation, deep breathing exercises, yoga, or spending time in nature. These practices can help reduce stress hormones and promote a sense of calm, which will have a positive impact on blood sugar levels.

3. **Seeking Support**: Managing blood sugar can be challenging, especially if you are dealing with emotional or psychological issues. So, don't hesitate to reach out for support from friends, family, or a healthcare professional. Talking about your feelings and concerns can help alleviate stress and provide valuable insights into coping strategies.

4. **Setting Realistic Goals**: It is essential to set realistic goals for blood sugar management and recognize that progress may not always be linear. Don't be too hard on yourself if you experience setbacks or fluctuations in your blood sugar levels. Instead, focus on making small, sustainable changes and celebrate your successes along the way.

5. **Building Resilience**: Building resilience is an important aspect of managing blood

sugar and overcoming emotional challenges. Resilience refers to the ability to adapt to stress and adversity, bounce back from setbacks, and maintain a positive outlook. Practicing gratitude, fostering social connections, and engaging in activities that bring you joy can help build resilience and enhance your overall well-being.

6. **Addressing Negative Thought Patterns**: Negative thought patterns, such as catastrophizing or all-or-nothing thinking, contribute to stress and anxiety and negatively impact blood sugar management. Challenge these negative thoughts by replacing them with more balanced and realistic perspectives. For example, instead of thinking, "I'll never be able to control my blood sugar," reframe it as, "I'm taking positive steps to manage my blood sugar, and I'm making progress."

7. **Incorporating Mindful Eating Practices**: Mindful eating involves paying attention to your food choices, eating slowly, and savoring each bite. By practicing mindful eating, you can become more attuned to your body's hunger and fullness cues, which will help prevent emotional eating and promote healthier blood sugar levels. Additionally, mindful eating will enhance your overall enjoyment of food and promote satisfaction.

8. **Staying Flexible and Adaptable**: Blood sugar management requires flexibility and adaptability, especially when faced with unexpected challenges or changes in routine. Instead of viewing setbacks as failures, see them as opportunities to learn and grow. You will navigate the ups and downs of blood sugar management with

resilience and confidence by staying flexible
and adapting to changing situations.

Chapter 9

Long-Term Strategies for Blood Sugar Health

In this chapter, we will explore actionable steps you can take to maintain your progress and navigate potential challenges along the way. From dietary modifications to lifestyle adjustments, each strategy is tailored to empower you on your path to long-term blood sugar health.

Please note that managing blood sugar is not a one-time endeavor but a lifelong commitment to your well-being. You can proactively safeguard your health and mitigate the risk of complications associated with unstable blood sugar levels by implementing these strategies diligently. Don't forget that small changes yield significant results.

Maintaining Motivation and Consistency

Maintaining motivation and consistency in managing your blood sugar levels is crucial for long-term success and optimal health. It is natural to experience fluctuations in motivation, but there are strategies you can implement to stay on track.

One key aspect of maintaining motivation is setting realistic and achievable goals. Start by breaking down your larger health objectives into smaller, manageable steps. For example, instead of aiming to completely overhaul your diet overnight, focus on making one healthy change at a time, such as adding more vegetables into your meals or swapping sugary snacks for healthier alternatives.

It is also important to remind yourself of the reasons why you want to improve your blood sugar levels. Whether it is to reduce your risk of developing diabetes, improve your energy levels, or simply feel better overall, keeping your motivations front and center will help keep you focused during challenging times.

Another effective strategy for maintaining motivation is to surround yourself with a supportive community. This could be friends, family members, or online support groups who share similar health goals and can provide encouragement, accountability, and advice when needed. Sharing your progress, setbacks, and successes with others will help you stay motivated and inspired to keep moving forward.

In addition to setting goals and seeking support, finding activities that you enjoy and that align with your health goals will also help you stay motivated and consistent. Whether it is trying out a new exercise class, experimenting with healthy recipes, or exploring mindfulness techniques like meditation or yoga, finding activities that bring you joy can make it easier to stick to your health routine in the long term.

Lastly, remember to be kind to yourself and practice self-compassion along the way. It is normal to experience setbacks and challenges on your health journey, but instead of getting discouraged, use these moments as opportunities for growth and learning. Celebrate your progress, no matter how small, and remember that every positive choice you make is a step in the right direction towards better blood sugar health and overall well-being.

Tracking Progress and Making Adjustments

Tracking your progress and making adjustments are crucial aspects of managing your blood sugar levels effectively. By closely monitoring your lifestyle habits and glucose readings, you will be able to identify areas for improvement and tailor your approach accordingly.

The following are strategies for tracking your progress and making necessary adjustments to support your long-term blood sugar health.

1. **Regular Glucose Monitoring**: One of the most important tools for tracking your progress is regular glucose monitoring. This involves checking your blood sugar levels at specific times throughout the day, such as before and after meals, before and after exercise, and at bedtime. By keeping a log of your glucose readings, you can identify

patterns and trends over time, allowing you to make informed adjustments to your diet, exercise routine, and medication regimen.

2. **Utilizing Technology**: In today's digital age, there are several technological tools available to help you track your blood sugar levels more effectively. From smartphone apps to wearable devices, these tools make it easier than ever to monitor your glucose levels and track your progress over time. Some apps even allow you to sync your glucose data with your healthcare provider. This enables them to provide personalized recommendations based on your individual needs.

3. **Keeping a Food Diary**: Another valuable tool for tracking your progress is keeping a food diary. By recording everything you eat and drink throughout the day, you can identify potential triggers for blood sugar spikes and make adjustments to your diet accordingly. Pay close attention to portion

sizes, carbohydrate content, and timing of meals and snacks, as these factors can all impact your blood sugar levels.

4. **Tracking Physical Activity**: Regular physical activity is a vital component of blood sugar management, but it is important to track your activity levels to ensure you are getting enough exercise without overexerting yourself. Keep a log of your daily activity, including the type, duration, and intensity of exercise, as well as any changes in your blood sugar levels before and after physical activity. This will help you identify the optimal exercise routine for maintaining stable blood sugar levels.

5. **Monitoring Medication and Supplement Use**: If you are taking medication or supplements to manage your blood sugar levels, it is important to monitor their effectiveness and adjust your dosage as needed. Keep track of when you take your

medications or supplements, as well as any changes in your blood sugar levels or overall health. Be sure to communicate with your healthcare provider about any concerns or questions you may have about your medication regimen.

6. **Seeking Support**: Managing blood sugar levels can be challenging, but you don't have to do it alone. Seek support from friends, family members, or a healthcare provider who can offer guidance, encouragement, and accountability. Consider joining a support group or online community for people with diabetes or blood sugar issues, where you can share experiences, ask questions, and learn from others who are on a similar journey.

7. **Adjusting Your Approach**: As you track your progress and make adjustments to your lifestyle habits, be prepared to experiment with different strategies to find what works best for you. What works for

one person may not work for another, so it is important to listen to your body and trust your instincts. Don't be afraid to try new foods, exercises, or medications, and be open to making changes as needed to achieve your blood sugar goals.

Celebrating Success and Staying Committed to Long-term Health Goals

Celebrating success and staying committed to long-term health goals is crucial for maintaining optimal blood sugar levels and overall well-being. As you continue on your journey towards better health, you should acknowledge and celebrate your achievements along the way. You will stay motivated and inspired to continue making positive choices for your health by recognizing your progress and accomplishments.

One way to celebrate success is by setting milestones for yourself. These milestones can be small, achievable goals that you work towards over time. For example, you might set a goal to exercise for 30 minutes each day or to incorporate more vegetables into your meals. When you reach these milestones, take the time to celebrate your achievement. This could involve treating yourself to a healthy meal at your favorite restaurant or rewarding yourself with a new workout outfit.

Another way to celebrate success is by sharing your achievements with others. Whether it is with friends, family, or members of a support group, sharing your progress will help keep you accountable and motivated. You might consider joining a social media group dedicated to blood sugar management where you can connect with others who are on a similar journey. You will gain valuable insights and support from others who understand what you are going through if you share your successes and challenges.

In addition to celebrating your own success, it is crucial to recognize the progress of others. By celebrating the achievements of those around you, you can create a supportive and encouraging environment that promotes growth and success for everyone involved. This could involve congratulating a friend who has reached their own health goals or offering words of encouragement to someone who is struggling. By lifting each other up, you will be creating a sense of community that fuels both motivation and commitment to long-term health goals.

As you celebrate your successes and stay committed to your long-term health goals, remember to stay focused on the bigger picture. While it is important to celebrate each milestone along the way, it is equally important

to maintain perspective and keep your
long-term goals in mind.

Conclusion

Empowering Yourself for Lifelong Blood Sugar Wellness

I congratulate you for making it to the pages of "Blood Sugar Solution Kit Book: The Complete Guide to Managing Your Blood Sugar - Essential Strategies, Recipes, and Tips for Optimal Health." I am glad that you have been empowered and equipped with the knowledge and tools to take control of your blood sugar levels and optimize your overall health for years to come.

If you implement the strategies outlined in this book, you will be able to make informed decisions about your diet, lifestyle, and overall health. Each chapter of this book has been carefully put together to provide you with actionable steps and valuable insights. Whether you are managing diabetes, striving for weight loss, or simply aiming to improve your overall health, the information presented here is relevant and applicable to your journey towards optimal wellness.

Let me remind you that the key to long-term success lies in consistency and commitment. By staying mindful of your choices and making small, sustainable changes over time, you will be able to achieve lasting results and enjoy a life filled with vitality and well-being.

Finally, I encourage you to stay curious, stay informed, and above all, stay empowered. With the knowledge and resources provided in this book, you have the power to take control of your blood sugar and live your best life.

Thank you for allowing me to be a part of your wellness journey. Here's to your health, happiness, and vitality.